Woman's World...

Simple ways to a beautiful life

Table of Contents

Introduction

Beauty is the aggregate of qualities in a person or thing that gives pleasure to the senses, mind, or spirit. – Merriam-Webster

Every woman wants to be beautiful: happy, healthy, independent, loved, and fulfilled. Sometimes, however, we do not have (or make) time to manage our lives so that we can achieve these goals. We are so busy dealing with the demands of the moment that we forget about our dreams. We think these dreams are not so important now—maybe tomorrow or next month or next year we will have time do something for ourselves.

If you are reading this, you have an opportunity to change your life. Seize this opportunity now—not tomorrow, next week, next month, or next year. Give yourself the gift of change right now. Take a few minutes to recall the dreams you once had. Revise those dreams if necessary; then visualize—in detail—the life you want. Now make a commitment to achieve that life by following a few simple steps that will energize both your body and spirit.

Use this book as a guide to help you understand the basics of good health, style, beauty (inner and outer), self-reliance, and self-esteem. Learn how to achieve your goals and how good money management will not only improve your finances but also reduce stress and enhance personal relationships. This little book is filled with ideas to help you become strong and happy, secrets that will lead to happiness and success in both the personal and professional aspects of your life.

This book is not only about how to be beautiful; it's also about how to recapture beauty and keep it through the years. It will help you discover your own unique path in life—a path filled with good health, confidence, happiness, and a youthful spirit.

Basics of a Healthy Lifestyle

The best six doctors anywhere
And no one can deny it
Are sunshine, water, rest, and air
Exercise and diet.
These six will gladly you attend
If only you are willing
Your mind they'll ease
Your will they'll mend
And charge you not a shilling.
~Nursery rhyme quoted by Wayne Fields, What the River Knows,
1990

To avoid sickness eat less; to prolong life worry less. ~
Chu Hui Weng

A healthy lifestyle incorporates all our daily habits and attitudes—from how much coffee we drink to how we deal with stress. Day or night, every choice we make either improves or impairs how we look and feel.

For many of us, a long, peaceful sleep is a luxury we simply do not always have time for. However, we must remember that getting enough high-quality sleep is one of the secrets of lifelong health and beauty. Fresh air in the bedroom promotes better sleep. Good sleep allows the body to re-energize. Both your muscles and your brain require periodic rest. Sleep specialists recommend going to bed before midnight and getting at least seven hours of sleep each night. The quality of sleep is equally important. Before falling asleep, try to let go of stressful thoughts or unresolved problems. Find something pleasant to focus on so you can relax and allow your body to rest peacefully.

Nutritious food is another key to youthful appearance and a longer, healthier life. Before eating salty snacks or sweet desserts, ask yourself, "Will this food support my health and beauty?" If the answer is "No," limit your portion or make a better choice. Unless you have a food-related medical condition, it is not necessary to follow a special diet; simply choose foods wisely (less meat, more fruits and vegetables) and enjoy them in moderation.

Do not forget to get some physical exercise every day. For example, use the stairs instead of the escalator or elevator. If possible, walk to work (or at least to the bus stop). Take a walk in the fresh air before sleeping. When you eat well, stay physically active, and get enough good sleep, you will look and feel your best.

There a lots of other little things—simple things—you can do to maintain good health and youthfulness. It is important to drink plenty of liquids, take vitamins every day, and avoid smoking (including second-hand smoke). Always use sunscreen with UVA protection on your face and hands to prevent premature aging of the skin and serious diseases such as a skin cancer.

It is also wise to have your blood pressure checked—keeping it under control may save your life (or at least extend it by many years). Have a yearly mammogram, and a full physical exam as often as your doctor recommends. Don't be afraid to ask questions; women must be advocates for their own health.

To stay emotionally healthy, never compare yourself to women from magazines or Hollywood. Every woman is unique, and unrealistic comparisons can lead to strong depression. (Besides, we never know what these women's lives are really like.) Do not subject yourself to unnecessary stress. Mental and emotional stress always has physical symptoms, affecting the condition of a skin, nails and hair, as well as influencing our general health and accelerating the aging process. If certain life situations create unavoidable stress, find healthy strategies (yoga, exercise, music, etc.) to manage it

Most importantly, enjoy life. Learn how to find something joyful in even the worst of days. The ability to relax, laugh and rejoice will prolong your life for many, many years.

Your Turn: *Keep a gratitude or joy journal. Use an inexpensive, pocket-size notebook or the computer. Each day, record at least one thing that made you laugh or smile, gave you a deeper sense of gratitude, or brought you joy. Record five of your favorite entries here.*

Step One: Nutrition

"Those who think they have no time for healthy eating will sooner or later have to find time for illness." – Edward Stanley

Eating well is the most important element in maintaining good health, good looks, and vitality. Food is our body's fuel, the energy source that gives us mobility and feeds our muscles and brain.

Everything we eat influences our health, the condition of our body, and its ability to function. Too much fat in our diet will increase the level of fat in hair and skin. On the contrary, a diet with too little fat will lead to thin nails, dry skin and fragile hair. Too little water causes the body to become dehydrated, which allows the accumulation of many toxins that can affect our overall health.

Balancing the types of food we eat is important. Our daily diet should include water, fiber, protein, carbohydrates, some fat, and lots of vitamins. Practicing good nutrition may require a change in lifestyle. One by one, you can replace bad eating habits with ones that support good health, foster a positive attitude, and fit the specific demands of your life. For example, if you get very hungry between meals, you should have something wholesome (fruit, herbal tea, or a small handful of nuts) nearby so that you can quickly and easily satisfy that hunger.

Food Pyramids

A well balanced diet is often represented in the form of a pyramid. The traditional pyramid includes five basic groups of foods distributed according to their importance for health. The foundation of this pyramid is water, as this is the most important element of any diet. Above water are whole grains, rice and pasta. Fruit and vegetables are next because they have fiber and lots of vitamins and minerals. Moving up the pyramid, the fourth group is proteins. The fifth group is comprised of fats, vegetable oils and sweets. This group takes up a very small part of the pyramid because we should limit fatty foods in our diet.

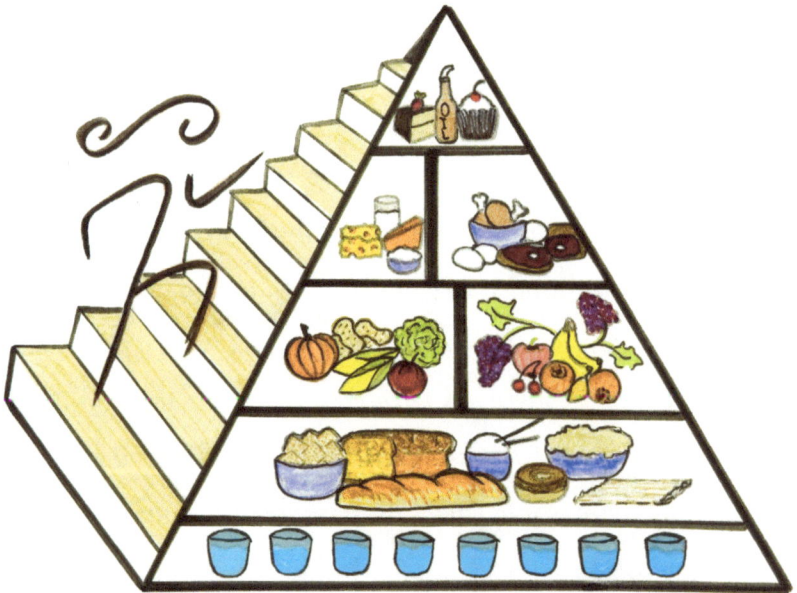

In 2005, the U.S. Department of Agriculture created a new pyramid that regrouped foods into a vertical spectrum of six groups and added an element of physical exercise. The USDA also developed twelve intake

profiles that suggest the proper ratio of food groups for specific types of individuals such as athletes, preschoolers, and new mothers.

The Value of Water

The most important thing we can do for our bodies is to drink plenty of water, at least eight glasses a day. Juice, soda, coffee and other drinks do not count, as they contain other ingredients such as caffeine, sugar, or sugar substitutes. If you do not enjoy plain water, add a few slices of lemon or lime. Water helps our body get rid of harmful substances that can poison it.

Be sensitive to your body's needs. If your mouth is dry, that is a signal that you need more water. Insufficient hydration causes thirst, headache, fatigue, and general physical deterioration. Lack of water also slows down our digestive process and decreases our ability to work efficiently.

Drink more water each day, beginning first thing in the morning. This will reduce hunger, clear your body of damaging substances, and give you more energy. Hot water with lemon in the morning also flushes toxins from your intestines.

Fruits and Vegetables

Fruits and vegetables are rich in nutrients and should constitute a major portion of our diet. They lower cholesterol, strengthen our immune system, remove toxins from the body, and slow down the aging process. As with any substance, their benefits are soaked up faster if they are eaten on an empty stomach; therefore, it is better to eat at least *some of these foods separately from other items. Fruit, for example, it is more beneficial if eaten on an empty stomach and at least half an hour before eating any other food.*

Vegetables are a powerful source of nutrition. Dark green, leafy vegetables such as kale, brussels sprouts, spinach, bok choy and broccoli are especially rich in fiber, Vitamin A, and antioxidants. (An antioxidant is a substance that protects cells from the damaging effects of free radicals. Free radicals are highly reactive chemicals that attach to cellular molecules such as DNA.) Yellow vegetables such as carrots, sweet potatoes, pumpkins and squash contain large amounts of beta-carotene, which converts to Vitamin A. Vitamin A is known to promote good eyesight and healthy, smooth skin. It may also help in preventing cancer.

It is interesting to note the role of peppers in a healthy diet. Sweet peppers are rich in Vitamin C, thiamine, Vitamin B6, beta carotene, and folic acid and have exceptional antioxidant activity. Peppers also *contain calcium, iron, phosphorus, and iodine.* They are helpful in protecting against cataracts and preventing cardiovascular and inflammatory diseases. Red bell peppers have significantly higher levels of nutrients than green and contain lycopene, which helps protect against cancer and heart disease. *The regular use of sweet pepper improves the condition of skin and hair, dilutes the blood, and stimulates appetite.*

Spicy red peppers contain large amounts of Vitamin C and beta-carotene. They strengthen the immune system, fight infection, regulate blood circulation and generally improve cardiovascular health. Black pepper isn't really a vegetable, but it is a powerful antioxidant.

The water in which vegetables are cooked is also very useful; it is rich with vitamins and easy to absorb. Be sure to wash vegetables before cooking them; after cooking, store the cooking water in the refrigerator and drink it when your stomach is empty. Eating fresh, raw vegetables (and fruits) can also supply some of your daily water needs.

Fruits also provide a wealth of nutrition. Nearly all berries (and especially blueberries) are full of antioxidants. Plums (and prunes) are also high in antioxidants, as well as vitamins A, C and K, and potassium. Plums increase our ability to absorb iron, improve digestion, protect eyesight, and strengthen immunity to some cancers. Citrus fruits are a great source of Vitamin C, as well as bioflavinoids (substances that strengthen blood vessels) and fiber. Apples and dates are also an excellent fiber source. Bananas, pomegranates and dates are good sources of potassium. Dates also promote good digestion, are rich in antioxidants, and contain several B-complex vitamins, which makes them a quick and effective energy booster. Eating more fruits and vegetables will not only keep you healthy, it will also make it easier to maintain a reasonable weight.

The Role of Fiber

Nutritionists recommend 25 to 35 grams of fiber per day for the average adult. Good sources of fiber include whole-grain breads and cereals, semolina pasta, brown rice, beans, nuts and seeds. Some fruits and vegetables, such as apples, pears and artichokes, also contain significant fiber. High-fiber foods naturally clean out the digestive system, removing toxins and irritants. Fiber contains vitamins and antioxidants, and has practically no calories. If you regularly include lots of fiber in your diet, you will have strong nails, pure skin, and healthy, shiny hair. If you increase your fiber intake, be sure to drink extra water to reduce digestive gasses.

Vitamins

A healthy diet must include vitamins A, C, D, E, folic acid, and the B-complex. The essential fatty acids Omega-3 and Omega-6 are also vital for healthy skin, hair and nails, as well as cell maintenance and support of numerous internal systems.

It is better to take multivitamins than a variety of special vitamins for nails, hair or skin. Multivitamins contain the full range of necessary vitamins, and special vitamins contain only certain group of vitamins. It is also important to remember that megadoses of any vitamin can be dangerous to your health.

The Truth about Chocolate

Some women think they cannot live without chocolate, and there is some chocolate they shouldn't live without. Very dark chocolate (at least 70% cacao) contains more antioxidants and less sugar than milk chocolate and provides several other nutritional benefits. It stimulates endorphins (natural pain relievers) and contains serotonin, a natural anti-depressant. Dark chocolate also strengthens our immune system, reduces cellular damage, and helps burn fat, regulate blood pressure and lower cholesterol. To get the most benefit, look for chocolate with the fewest additives.

Foods to Avoid

Avoid fried food and food that has passed through thermal processing. Thermally processed foods may contain poisonous gasses that deprive your body of its natural ability to dispose of the processing products. Retention of these gasses can affect metabolism, digestion, the condition of hair, skin and nails, and general health.

Use fresh foods whenever possible, refrigerating or otherwise storing items appropriately. When using frozen or canned foods, always check expiration dates. Frozen foods cannot be kept indefinitely. If too much ice builds up on the surface of a frozen item, it will lose its flavor and nutrition.

When using canned or other ready-to-eat foods, always read the labels carefully. Try to buy products that have fewer than ten ingredients. Avoid products that include ingredients you can't pronounce or have never heard of.

A healthy diet limits consumption of carbonated drinks, beer and other alcoholic beverages, as well as salt, sugar, sugar substitutes, and caffeine, which dehydrate the body and accelerate aging.

Do not overeat! Limit snacks and keep them healthy. And always include lots of water and fiber in your diet because these help cleanse your internal systems.

Digestion

Good digestion promotes a cheerful disposition. Therefore, make an effort to eat in a relaxed environment and take time to thoroughly chew your food. As mentioned above, drink plenty of water, and eat fruit and other foods rich in fiber. Adding cinnamon to drinks or food can improve peristalsis, the wavelike contractions of your digestive system.

So many aspects of good health depend on the condition of your digestive system. If any aspect of your digestive process concerns you, consult your doctor—and don't be afraid to ask questions.

Weight Loss and Health

Whenever losing weight is necessary, it becomes even more important to focus on healthy eating. It is impossible to lose weight or see an improvement in health unless you make reasonable and consistent changes in your eating habits. If you follow an extreme diet that doesn't include a balance of foods or that limits your daily intake to less than 1000 calories, you will probably lose weight too fast. Such extreme diets can also damage your heart, liver, or other internal organs. Studies also show that women who lose weight too quickly are very likely to gain it all back, sometimes gaining even more weight than they lost.

Avoid using diet supplements to lose weight, because they can damage your health. Instead, eat well, be active every day, and give yourself time for rest and recreation. Daily intake of a variety of healthy foods, lots of water, and multivitamins is the key to long-lasting health and beauty.

Your Turn: Choose one commitment you are ready to make to keep yourself healthy and full of vitality. Be specific. Be realistic. Write your commitment.

Beauty Basics

Pretty is something you're born with. But beautiful,
that's an equal opportunity adjective. – author unknown

Beauty is reflected in sparkling eyes, a charming smile, light step, and pleasant voice. Many books have been written about beauty secrets, but the most fundamental truth is no secret at all: beauty requires daily work. Good nutrition is the foundation, but to remain youthful and attractive for many years, women also need to learn and practice the basics of proper daily care of the face, hair, skin, hands, feet, and nails.

A Radiant Face

A woman's most important feature is her face. Unfortunately, many of us realize too late that smooth, beautiful skin does not last forever without gentle care. Facial skin needs to be cleansed, moisturized, nourished and protected daily.

Our face is constantly exposed to external influences. Though the sun is a wonderful source of Vitamin D, it is also the primary cause of damage to the skin. Therefore it is necessary to use a cream with UVA protection, even in the winter or on cloudy days. Daily use of UVA protection is really important because UVA rays not only increase the likelihood of skin cancer, they also destroy the natural collagen in our skin, drying the skin and creating wrinkles.

The face requires constant and careful attention. Always be sure your hands are clean before you touch your face. If possible, try not to touch it at all during the day. Do not scratch the skin with your nails. Never rub your face, as rubbing damages skin cells and leads to the formation of wrinkles. Treat the skin on your face as gently as you would treat a baby's skin.

To care for your face properly, it is necessary to first find out what type of skin you have, and then to use products designed specifically for that type. You can determine your skin type with the help of a professional or by yourself. To define skin type on your own, first wash your face thoroughly. Two or three hours later, place a clean paper napkin on your forehead, another on your nose and chin, and a third on your cheek. If oil traces appear on the napkins, your skin is oily. If traces only appear on the forehead, nose and chin, your skin is a combination of oily and normal. If no traces appear, your skin is normal. Another way to check is to press a finger on your skin. If the impression disappears at once, the skin is normal; if the impression remains, the skin is dry. Remember, for either of these tests to be accurate, your skin must be absolutely clean.

It is very important to remove make-up every night, using cool water and gentle gels or face washes. Soap dries the skin, so it is not recommended. Products identified as make-up removers are best because they do not irritate the skin but they do moisturize it. Except for the area around your eyes, baby wipes are good make-up removers. They contain special lotion which both cleans and moisturizes the skin. Even if you don't wear make-up, it is necessary to clean and moisturize your face before sleeping in order to remove dirt and airborne impurities that can cause blackheads or other blemishes.

If you use a night cream, you must wash your face again in the morning to clear your pores. Otherwise, it is enough simply to rinse your face with cool water in the morning.

To maintain elasticity in your skin, regularly use nourishing or moisturizing face masks, a rich night cream, and a day moisturizer with UVA protection. If you use lotion, choose one with a non-alcohol base. Alcohol dries the skin, depriving it of the natural oils that give it a healthy glow. If you have oily skin, choose a lighter, less oily cream or use a moisturizing lotion that is easily absorbed. If your skin is dry, an oil-based cream is recommended. To restore skin to a fresh, healthy, radiant condition, I recommend scrubs, masks or peels that remove dead skin and open pores.

If the weather becomes exceptionally hot, moisturizers can be stored in the refrigerator. This maintains the integrity of ingredients and makes application of the product more refreshing. If creams become too cold, rub the container between your palms to warm it; this allows the skin to absorb the cream more easily. Try to apply cream at least twenty minutes prior to leaving the house so it has time to be absorbed.

Never squeeze blemishes on your face. This can lead to the formation of scars or damage underlying layers of a skin. If you frequently have facial blemishes or inflammation, you may not be cleaning your face well enough, or you have a habit of touching it with dirty hands, or you may simply need to change your pillowcase more often. If the problem persists, you should discuss it with your doctor.

If you have access to a sauna, it can be very helpful to your skin. The heat improves blood circulation and brings nutrients to the face. It *softens the skin and creates a healthy radiance that makes us look younger. Before entering a sauna, clean your face thoroughly and apply a moisturizer to protect it from the hot steam.*

Twice a month you may want to give your face a deeper cleansing with a facial sauna. This will clear your skin of oil, toxins, and external impurities. Create aromatic steam by steeping one or two tablespoons of rose petals, chamomile, or birch leaves in a quart of water. Pour the boiling water into a bowl and hold a towel over your head so the steam flows directly into your face. Keep steam on your face for 3-10 minutes, depending on your skin type. (Generally, allow about three minutes for dry skin, five for combination, and ten for oily.) After the steam, use a scrub appropriate for your skin type on the face and neck, applying it with gentle circular movements. After rinsing the scrub, smooth on lotion to prevent irritation.

Before discussing the proper care of other parts of the body, it is important to note that the skin of the neck and décolleté areas requires the same constant, gentle care as the face. Otherwise, your face may say you are thirty, but your neck may look more like forty.

Do not worry about the money you spend on skin care products. As long as you are actually using the products, they will not only correct faults, but also nourish the skin and protect it from external damage.

Enchanting Eyes

Because the skin around our eyes is very thin and lacks collagen, it requires very gentle care. Without special care, this area of the face may make us appear much older than we really are.

It is necessary to use products designed especially for care of skin around the eyes. These products will slow down the aging process by protecting the skin from irritants and toxins in the environment. Since exposure to sun is the most common aging factor, always choose an eye cream with UVA protection.

Apply cream to eyelids with gentle, circular movements of your ring finger, the weakest finger of a hand. Do not rub the cream in; it will be absorbed on its own. Never stretch the skin either. Improper care of skin around the eyes leads to early wrinkles, so always be careful when you attend to this area.

Again, it is important to purchase high quality cosmetics for the eyes. Inferior products can injure the surface of your eye and even lead to deterioration or loss of sight. Replace mascara every three months; otherwise, bacteria develop that can lead to inflammation of the eyelids. Apply mascara carefully to avoid damaging the surface of the eye or causing infection. Eye shadows and pencils should only be used for about six months. Avoid touching eye pencils or other eye make-up with your tongue; saliva may encourage the formation of bacteria in cosmetics, and that bacteria may cause a serious eye infection.

Eyes attract attention, so we want to emphasize them when applying make-up. For daytime, it is better to use shades similar to natural skin tones. In an evening, however, you can use darker, more dramatic colors and even a light touch of glitter for a special occasion.

To remove eye make-up, always use products designed for the eyes. High quality olive oil or children's Vaseline can also be used. Again, be careful not to rub the skin and, to prevent infection, be sure to remove all eye make-up every night. To reduce wrinkles, put a few drops of olive or almond oil under your eyes just before going to sleep. Keep these oils in the refrigerator to preserve the Vitamin E. You can also break a Vitamin E capsule and dab the oil onto the skin around your eyes.

Never use an astringent or alcohol-based product near the eyes. These are harmful to eyelids and dangerous to eyes.

Eyebrows are another important part of the face. Use tweezers to shape them, or have a professional beautician shape and/or color them for you. Check eyebrows regularly so they do not become overgrown. (Women past menopause may find their eyebrows thinning and should use a good-quality pencil to fill them in.)

Luscious Lips

The skin on our lips is also very thin and easily injured, so it needs constant, careful attention. Regular use of your favorite lip balm will help prevent cracks, supply nutrients, and provide some antiseptic protection.

To keep lips soft, it is necessary to remove dead or dry skin. This can be done by gently massaging them with a moistened, soft-bristle toothbrush or a clean, damp piece of a soft cloth such as terry. There are also special lip peels, which should be used very carefully. Never bite or tear off bits of dry skin from the lips; this can cause more serious damage or infection.

Before beginning your make-up routine, hydrate your lips with moisturizer. Apply lipstick or gloss as the last step in the make-up process. Use a brush to apply lipstick; it will be easier to distribute the color evenly and accurately. If you want lipstick to last longer, outline the lips with a lipstick pencil first. Frequent use of waterproof lipstick dries the lips. Using a gloss will make the lips more seductive.

Two final thoughts on lip care: When choosing lipstick or gloss, never put testers directly on the lips; only on the back of your hand. Also, before going to sleep each night, hydrate lips with a good moisturizer.

A Healthy Mouth

It is very important to take good care of both teeth and gums. Good oral health has been proven to influence the overall health of the body. Teeth need to be cleaned at least two times a day. (Cleaning the teeth before a breakfast will also freshen your breath and brighten your smile.)

Use dental floss and a good quality toothbrush. Replace the toothbrush every three to six months.

At your next dental check-up, ask the hygienist to show you how to clean your teeth correctly. Even though we have been brushing since we were toddlers, statistics show that most adults do not brush correctly. We attack the teeth, often with too much force or too stiff a toothbrush, and end up destroying enamel and injuring gums.

It is also a good idea to strengthen teeth and gums with a rinse or mouthwash. These not only promote fresh breath, they also protect teeth and gums from bacteria. To create a brighter smile, use a whitening toothpaste. Before choosing a tooth whitener, however, it is a good idea to talk to your dentist. Some whiteners can damage tooth enamel, which weakens the tooth and increases sensitivity. If you have sensitive enamel, look for toothpastes created specifically to reduce this problem.

Luxurious Hair

Hair is one of the first things people notice when they see us. Hair should always be clean and healthy. Daily shampooing is common and is recommended for oily hair or hair that is exposed to a lot of environmental pollutants. Curly hair may get too fluffy if washed every day. As with make-up and facial cleansers, always use high quality products formulated specifically for your type of hair. Drinking plenty of water and taking vitamins (particularly a B-complex supplement) will give your hair natural luster and vitality.

Earlier I mentioned that many of us don't know how to brush our teeth properly. The same is true for washing our hair. We've done it thousands of times, but perhaps have never done it correctly. First of all, it is a good idea to comb the hair through before washing. For washing, warm water, not hot, is recommended. Warm water opens the cuticle (covering) of the hair shaft to release oil and dirt; hot water does the same thing, but it also strips moisture from the hair and scalp. If you don't wash your hair every day, it is a good idea to shampoo twice. The first lather cleanses the hair of product and/or pollutants, and the second lather will enrich the scalp and hair follicles with nutrients.

Shampoo should be rubbed on the palms, then onto the scalp and gently worked out to the tips of each strand of hair. Massage the scalp with the balls of your fingers, using a circular motion. Do not let fingernails scrape the scalp; they can damage the skin or injure hair follicles.

After rinsing out the shampoo, be sure to apply a good conditioner. This will remove any residual shampoo, nourish the hair, facilitate combing, and make hair softer, smoother, and shiny. Regular use of conditioner will also protect hair from solar damage and the effects of chemicals in some styling products. To increase the benefits of the conditioner, towel dry your hair before applying; if conditioner is applied directly on wet hair, it will not be absorbed well and most of it will be washed away when you rinse. Lift hair with your fingers and work conditioner down from the ends toward the scalp. Never put conditioner directly on the scalp; over time it can penetrate and cause hair to age prematurely. Before rinsing, draw a wide-toothed comb through the hair so it will absorb more of the conditioning agent. Do this carefully so you don't irritate the hair or scalp. Finally, rinse hair with cool water. This closes the cuticle, adds shine to the hair, and stimulates blood circulation in the scalp.

Towel dry—gently pressing sections of hair between layers of towel—before styling. Do not rub or twist hair, as this damages the structure and causes split ends. Wet hair cannot be combed right away; first brush it with a soft brush. Then use your fingers to divide it into sections and comb each section with a wide-toothed comb. If you still have difficulty, use a good detangling conditioner or spray. This will protect the hair from damage as well as facilitate the combing process.

If you have trouble styling your hair, ask your hairdresser to teach you the process, step by step. Then you can have perfectly styled hair whenever you want, without spending a lot of money or taking time for a trip to the salon. If you must use a blow dryer to style your hair, keep it on low heat and use it as little as possible. Allow hair to dry naturally if possible.

Always think about your hair when you change environments. For example, if you are going to swim in a pool or relax in a hot tub, protect your hair from chlorine by dampening it first with cool water that will tighten the outer layer of each strand. If you will be swimming in salt water, use a conditioner designed for protection against salts. Avoid exposing hair (especially wet hair) to cold temperatures. If you visit a sauna, consider using the heat to enhance your hair as well. Apply a nourishing conditioner, and then cover the hair with a plastic cap and towel. The steam and increased temperature will allow your hair to absorb more of the conditioning agents. Finally, use a soft hair band to keep hair away from the face when applying or removing cosmetics.

If you want to color your hair, it is best to have this done by a professional. If you choose to do it yourself, at least seek professional advice regarding which products are best for your type of hair. Also be sure to regularly touch up the roots and trim dry or split ends. Otherwise, your hair will not have a well-groomed appearance.

Never make sudden changes to your hair. If you decide to dramatically change the color, cut or style, always give yourself a few days to think this idea through. If you don't, any "second thoughts" may come too late and you could be very unhappy.

Soft, Smooth Skin

As women, we also want beautiful skin all over our body. To keep skin soft and smooth, it is important to use a moisturizing lotion after every bath or shower. During pregnancy it is also necessary to use a nourishing cream, especially one with a high percentage of collagen, to prevent stretch marks.

As mentioned above, steam can be very beneficial to our skin. It improves blood circulation and helps rid the skin of impurities. After steam has opened up the pores, it is also good to use a body scrub or peel. Once or twice a week is often enough for this procedure. Before shaving, it is also wise to use steam or a commercial product to lift the hairs and protect the skin from irritation. Self-tanning lotions and sprays are currently very popular, but it is important to know how to apply these correctly. Always use an exfoliant first so the self-tanning product is applied to pure, dry skin. Avoid oil-based scrubs like shea butter, however, as they will cause the tanning colorant to be absorbed more deeply. For the same reason, it is necessary to moisturize drier skin (at elbows and knees, for example) before applying the tanner.

Many women today are concerned about cellulite. While there is no cure for this condition, there are several ways to reduce cellulite and improve appearance. At the first sign of a problem, check the Internet for information on the pros and cons of various massages, creams, and scrubs. (Some effective homemade scrubs can be made from instant coffee or coffee grounds.) Skin peels are also helpful, and tanning (natural or with product) will help disguise cellulite.

Youthful Hands, Beautiful Nails

It is often said that a woman's age can be determined by looking at her hands. And it is certainly true that the skin on our hands needs the most care, as it is exposed to more external damage than any other part of the body. To avoid premature wrinkles on the hands, first make a habit of always wearing work gloves when cleaning, washing dishes, or working in the garden. Also be sure to regularly moisturize hands with a high-quality hand cream or lotion. This not only keeps the skin soft, but also heals scratches and cracks that can be painful. Apply cream after every contact with water. Keep lotion near every sink, in your handbag, and on your beside table. Finally, when the weather is cold, be sure to wear gloves and apply lotion each time you come inside again. Rub lotion into nails and cuticle too; they require as much nourishment and hydration as your skin.

Everyone notices a woman's fingernails. They need not be fancy, but they should always be well groomed. Do not bite nails or cuticles; this can damage the nail root and growth cycle. Never use a fingernail as a tool; this will harm the nail structure. To keep hands looking well-groomed, have a regular manicure. Nail salons are very popular and relatively inexpensive, but you can also do a good manicure yourself. Be sure to disinfect all manicure accessories to prevent any chance of infection.

Begin the manicure by placing the hands in steam or in a mixture of liquid soap and lemon juice. Use cuticle softener and an orange stick to push the cuticle back. Before applying polish, be sure nails should are dry and free of oil so the polish will last longer. If you are using a strong color, carefully apply the polish evenly from the center to the edges of each nail. Avoid getting any polish on the skin, or quickly remove it with a dab of remover on a cotton swab. Poorly applied polish is far less attractive than no polish at all.

Chemical substances and soap weaken nails. Liquid polish remover should not be used more than twice a month. Special nourishing creams and nail strengtheners are available in drugstores, but the most important thing you can do for your nails is to eat well and drink plenty of water. (And, contrary to popular folklore, gelatin will not strengthen or improve the health of nails. Brittle nails are usually due to lack of moisture, not lack of protein.)

Sexy Feet

Every woman loves beautiful shoes. Beautiful shoes deserve beautiful feet. Even if you do not like your feet, it is very important to care for them. At the end of each day, try to make time for a foot soak, massage, or simple application of a cooling cream or gel. Products containing peppermint oil are especially refreshing for the feet.

To keep feet looking well groomed, remove any unnecessary or unsightly hair, use a pumice stone or similar device to smooth heels, and apply a nourishing or hydrating cream. A pedicure adds a nice finishing touch. A professional pedicure is especially good because it includes a soothing foot soak and/or massage. Professional care also helps prevent ingrown nails, nail fungus, and athlete's foot.

Fresh and Fragrant

A woman's scent is very important. The most essential element is cleanliness. The smell of pure, clean skin (with perhaps a lingering hint of fragrant cleanser) is exhilarating. Of course, it is also necessary to use a deodorant daily. Applied to clean skin, a good deodorant will keep you feeling fresh all day.

For many women, this clean, fresh smell is enough. Others prefer to personalize their scent with perfume. "Personalize" is the important word. Choose your scent carefully, paying attention to the comments and compliments of friends, but ultimately choosing the fragrance that is most pleasant to you. Try a variety of scents, using samplers from magazines or testers in stores, and be prepared to spend time doing a serious search before making a purchase.

To wear perfume well, it is helpful to understand its composition. All perfumes have four essential ingredients: alcohol, oils, water, and an aromatic infusion that defines the fragrance. The intensity and duration of a fragrance depend on the ratio of aromatic oils to solvent. Exact amounts vary with each manufacturer. Perfume averages approximately 20-30% aromatic infusion and eau de parfum about 15-20%. Toilet water (eau de toilette) provides the lightest scent, with 6-12% aromatic infusion. Perfume will retain its fragrance throughout the day, eau de parfum generally lasts four to five hours, and toilet water may only last an hour or so.

Perfume needs to be applied correctly so the aroma will envelope you as long as possible. Dab a drop or two on pulse spots—wrists, temples, inside elbows and knees, and behind the ears. Do not rub wrists together after applying fragrance; friction damages the chemical composition of the perfume, causing the aroma to fade more quickly. Using lotion with a similar fragrance will lengthen the amount of time before the aroma fades. Keeping perfume in a refrigerator will prolong its life, and perfume in a spray bottle will hold its fragrance longer because air has less access to the liquid.

Simple Routines

Even though there are hundreds of beauty tips and products, daily care really isn't very difficult. Simply remember that you are a fine woman whose body deserves as much nurturing as your mind and soul. Following a simple daily routine will prolong youth and enhance both inner and outer beauty.

Begin every morning with a smile. Hum your favorite song as you shower and wash your face. Apply deodorant, brush teeth, and quickly rub in a body cream. Dab the appropriate creams under eyes and on your face and neck. Apply perfume and lip balm. Do your make-up, style your hair, and get dressed. Once these procedures become a habit, they should take no more than 10-15 minutes. Your confidence and well-being are worth at least fifteen minutes, so be sure to reserve this time for yourself

Ahead of you a wonderful day awaits. Enjoy it.

Your Turn: Make the list of the cosmetics you need to properly care for hair, face, and body. Draw up a simple, daily self-care plan. Once you are comfortable with the daily routine, begin adding special treatments *to your schedule (for example, a face pack on Mondays, body scrub on Wednesdays, etc.—the next chapter offers recipes for many of these treatments). Post the schedule where you will see it every day.*

Beauty Recipes

For the Face

If your skin type is normal...

A simple olive oil mask will smooth wrinkles and soften and hydrate the skin. Wash your face thoroughly; then apply a thin layer of high-quality olive oil. Using a bowl of steaming water (not uncomfortably hot) and a towel over your head, let the steam saturate pores for 10-15 minutes. Afterwards, wipe any remaining oil from the face with a clean washcloth. This procedure is recommended every two weeks.

High-quality baby creams are also good for the face. For a quick moisturizing treatment, apply a thick layer of cream on a clean face for 20-30 minutes. Remove excess cream with a clean, wet cloth. Because these creams generally include an antiseptic, they may be used even if the skin is inflamed (but not on broken skin).

If your skin type is normal to dry...

An oatmeal mask will soften dry skin and improve your complexion. Soak about two ounces of old-fashioned oatmeal in two tablespoons of cream and two teaspoons honey. When the oatmeal has absorbed some of the liquid, the mixture will thicken and you can apply it to your face. Leave the mask on for twenty minutes and then wash it off with cool water.

If your skin is dry...

A honey and yogurt mask will nourish and hydrate dry skin. Combine equal amounts of honey and plain yogurt (no additives). Leave on the face for 20 minutes and then wash off with cool water.

An avocado mask is also excellent for dry skin. Combine one tablespoon of smashed avocado with a teaspoon of honey and a little sesame or olive oil. Leave the mask in place for ten minutes, and then wash it off with warm water.

If your skin is dry and sensitive...

Milk masks are very good for sensitive skin. Soak a clean cotton cloth in warm milk. Squeeze out excess liquid and place the cloth loosely over the face for ten minutes. When the cloth is removed, rinse your face well with warm water.

If your skin is normal to oily...

A calming and clarifying scrub is made of oatmeal and chamomile tea. To ¼ cup tea, add four tablespoons of old-fashioned oatmeal, two tablespoons honey and two drops almond oil. Mix well and rub gently onto face, neck, and décolleté area. Leave in place for 10-15 minutes and wash off with warm water.

If your skin is oily...

"Cleopatra's" egg white mask is remarkable. Beat an egg white until foamy. Spread over clean skin and leave in place for 15-20 minutes. Wash face with cool water. The egg white will shrink pores and nourish the skin, leaving it fresh and radiant.

Whatever type of skin you have...

Almond oil contains a high percentage of Vitamin E. Use it to remove eye make-up or as the basis of a face mask.

Olive oil is good for the skin. Make a mixture of olive oil, honey, and an egg yolk. Leave it on the face for twenty minutes, and then wash off with warm water.

A clay mask will help restore freshness and improve skin tone. Combine cosmetic clay (available at most drugstores) and water in a 1:2 ratio. (If skin is very dry, use milk instead of water.) You may also add honey and aromatic herbs such as peppermint or lavender. Apply the mask to clean skin, leave for 15 minutes, and then wash with cool water.

Toothpaste will minimize blemishes. Apply a small amount overnight to reduce inflammation. Repeat if necessary. A dab of clay mask also works.

Cucumber is good for eyelids. Place a freshly sliced piece over each closed eye and leave in place for ten minutes.

Olive oil will soften dry lips. It can be used alone or as part of a citrus scrub. To make the scrub, mix ½ teaspoon olive oil and ½ teaspoon honey; add one teaspoon granulated sugar and a few drops of lemon juice. Use a soft brush to gently rub the mixture over your lips.

Vaseline can be used to remove peeling skin from chapped lips. Apply a thin layer with a very soft brush and carefully rub over lips.

For the Body

Use Lemon to soften rough skin on elbows, knees and heels. Cut a lemon in half. Gently rub over problem zones and leave for 2-3 minutes. Then wash with cool water and soap and apply moisturizer. Repeat every 10-14 days as needed.

An oil and sugar scrub is also good for rough skin. Mix two tablespoons of olive oil and two tablespoons of granulated sugar. Apply to the body in gentle, circular motions, paying special attention to problem spots. Wash off with warm water.

A milk and oatmeal scrub will exfoliate dead skin. Mix milk, old-fashioned oats and baking soda until the mixture has the consistency of sour cream. After scrubbing, wash and dry skin and apply a good moisturizer.

A coffee scrub can reduce cellulite. Apply a thick paste of coffee grounds. Apply in circular motions on steamy hot skin. Rinse off with cool water to close pores.

Oatmeal and water makes a very simple, high-quality body scrub. Mix four parts water to one part old-fashioned oatmeal.

Honey and coarse salt also make an effective scrub. The salt exfoliates dead skin, and the honey nourishes remaining skin.

For Hair

Mayonnaise contains oils and nutrients that make hair healthier. Before going to bed, use your fingers to work a small amount of mayonnaise into hair. (Short hair may only need a teaspoon or two.) Cover your head with some plastic cap and a scarf and leave it in place overnight. In the morning, wash the mayonnaise out with warm water and shampoo. (If an overnight treatment is not possible, cover hair with a plastic cap for at least 40 minutes). Leaving mayonnaise (or any deep conditioner) on the hair overnight is much more effective than a 40-minute treatment. To avoid making hair oily, do not use this treatment more than once a week.

Olive oil nourishes the scalp and strengthens hair. Mix one teaspoon of olive oil with a small amount of lemon juice and two egg yolks. Work the mixture into hair and cover with a plastic cap for 30-40 minutes. Wash the mixture out with warm or cool water.

A similar mixture uses three tablespoons of olive oil, 2 ounces of honey, and one egg. Leave mixture on hair for 20 minutes, and then wash out with shampoo.

An infusion of mint, chamomile, or young nettles in rinse water will also improve the structure of hair strands.

Honey and egg yolk will nourish and repair dry hair. Combine two tablespoons honey and three beaten egg yolks. Apply the mixture to hair and scalp and leave for 30 minutes. Cover hair with a plastic cap for another 30-40 minutes, then rinse thoroughly with cool water. This can be done as often as you like.

For very dry or damaged hair, apply this mixture (or any conditioner) for 20 minutes before washing.

Coconut oil *is very good for the scalp. It can be used alone or mixed with honey (two parts oil to one part honey) before gently rubbing onto the skin. Leave for 30 minutes, then wash out with shampoo. Massaging the scalp with warm oils will also improve the condition of dry hair.*

Apple vinegar or lemon juice *can give your hair more shine. Use about one tablespoon of either per each quart of water.*

Your Turn: *Choose five recipes that especially interest you. List them below. Try one each week and write yourself a reminder of how well it worked (or didn't), what you might do differently, etc.*

Motion is Life

Movement is a medicine for creating change in a person's physical, emotional, and mental states. – Carol Welch

Our body has been created for motion. Movement stimulates the heart, mind and soul. Regular physical activity not only positively influences physical health; it also affects our mental and emotional state. Physical activity burns fat and calories, stimulates blood circulation, tones muscles, clears the body of toxins through sweat, and generally slows down the aging process. When a woman is physically active, her figure and energy level improve, which increases her self-esteem and self-confidence.

Physical exercise is very effective when done in the morning on an empty stomach. For the best results, try to exercise for at least thirty minutes each day. Work hard enough to get your pulse rate up, but not so hard that you can't talk comfortably while you are moving. If you do not have time to participate in a sport, it is a good idea to invest in some exercise equipment; otherwise you may end up with flabby thighs or a big behind. No matter what time or type of exercise you choose, your body will adjust and respond if you are consistent.

Experts differ on whether there's a best time to exercise. Many people prefer to work out first thing in the morning because there are no distractions. Others prefer late afternoon because the exercise relieves stress. What's really important is that, whatever time of day you choose, you stick with it, exercising for at least thirty minutes five times a week.

Whatever your level of activity, it's good to begin every morning with some stretching and light calisthenics, which are both pleasant and useful. These will help your body wake up and improve overall muscle tone. Play your favorite music, and always smile while you exercise. If the routine becomes boring, try some new music and remind yourself that flexibility, strength and endurance are necessary for good health and a long and youthful life.

To maintain good health, stay active, engage in any sport or sports of your choosing, and get lots of fresh air. (One caution: It is always wise to have a physical and consult with a doctor before taking up any new sport. Otherwise, you may incur unnecessary injury.) Above all, choose activities that you enjoy. It won't be long before you realize that regular physical activity does make you stronger, healthier and more self-assured.

Your Turn: *Think about your current physical activity. What activity involves you most of all? Perhaps it is dance or simply walking. What activity would you like to do more? Choose one and create a reasonable plan to include it in your daily/weekly schedule.*

Dressing with Style

Fashions fade. Style is eternal.   – Yves Saint Laurent

Today's world places a lot of value on style. Every woman enjoys dressing well and feeling beautiful, but not all attempts at style turn out well. Some women strive to create their own unique style; others follow fashion trends carefully so their style is always current; and others simply put on whatever is clean and comfortable because they're afraid they may look silly if they try to be stylish or they believe that style requires a huge expense.

In truth, learning to dress well can be a lot of fun for women. There's no reason to be nervous or to spend huge sums of money for clothes and accessories. All you really need is imagination and some common sense. For example, your daughter's (or mother's) sweater may look beautiful with your own slacks. You can also borrow a sister's necklace or a friend's skirt. Visit consignment shops to find high-end clothing at reasonable prices. Add unique items to your wardrobe by making or decorating them yourself. Knit or crochet a sweater, make a beautiful bead bracelet, or to sew sequins on your jeans. Save time by planning in advance (for example, while preparing a meal) how you wish to look.

Choose clothes that you love and wear them with pleasure. Feeling confident in your clothes is the basis of success in any business. You only get one body in this life—love it, take care of it, and dress it well.

Bearing

Our bearing—posture and the physical mannerisms that reflect personality and attitude—determines the first impression we give others. At a correct bearing, the chin forms a right angle with the body, shoulders are straightened, and the stomach is tightened. This position is the most natural, as pressure on the backbone is distributed at regular intervals. Keep your head up and maintain visual contact when talking with others. Proper bearing not only adds grace to your figure, it also allows internal organs to work most efficiently. Poor posture pushes the head in front of the body, increasing the relative weight of the head by a factor of ten with each inch forward. The long-term effects of improper bearing include discomfort, pain, and possible disability.

Personal Style

Think carefully about what style is best for you. Sketch, cut out pictures, or simply describe in writing how you wish to look. Include clothes, accessories, and hairstyle. Begin with an honest assessment of your face and figure, and concentrate on the positive aspects as you develop your style.

Learn to choose clothes that emphasize your best features and hide the less becoming ones. If you have beautiful breasts, long feet, lovely shoulders or a narrow waist, wear clothes that draw the eye toward these. Try on lots of clothes until you begin to understand what type of neckline, skirt, jacket, trouser, or jeans suits your best. Once you figure out what styles and colors are most flattering, you will always look good. Whether it's a business suit, a sexy evening dress, or casual attire for a sporting event, always choose items that fit well and are comfortable. Also be alert to appropriate ways to add a splash of color or texture, as these add interest to an outfit.

Following these guidelines, you will soon develop a style that expresses your personality, enhances your confidence, and leads you to success.

Clothing Basics

Always try clothes on before buying. Just because a certain style of jeans sits well on your girlfriend does not mean they will sit the same way on you. And never assume a piece of clothing will fit properly because it's the "right" size. Most women have a range of at least three sizes, depending on the style and type of garment. What's important is the fit and flatter of the style, not the number on the label. After you get home, you can always cut off the size number.

The clothes you choose should not only fit well, but also be comfortable. Consider natural fabrics such as cotton, silk, cashmere and wool that allow your skin to breathe. Nothing should irritate or constrict the body. Clothes that are too tight can restrict the flow of blood. Skinny jeans, for example, may be a factor in the development of blood clots, as well as yeast infections and reduced bowel function. Finally, if any clothing leaves deep purple stripes on your body give it to a friend or donate it to charity.

Fortunately, the days of boring, unattractive underwear are over. Now it is possible to purchase high-quality, comfortable lingerie *that is both beautiful and figure-enhancing—not rubbery and breath-constricting. A properly chosen bra can significantly change your life for the better. Most women do not wear the correct size or type of bra, so it's best to seek the help of a professional fitter. If the bra is too tight, it will create unsightly lines under clothing and may also impact the function of internal organs. If it is too large, or does not provide sufficient support, what good is it? Under light-colored fitted clothing, a nude shade of undergarment is preferable to white.*

When purchasing jeans, consider how their length corresponds to the type of footwear you prefer. The same jeans won't work with ballet flats and stiletto heels. With high heels, most women prefer jeans that "break" across the instep and fall somewhere between mid-heel and just above the floor in the back.

Keep clothes fresh and clean, always paying attention to specific laundering instructions. Attend to sewing repairs and stains immediately. (Be especially careful when putting on clothes after applying deodorant. Pull sweaters over the head first, then slip your arms into the sleeves.) Use good-quality hangers and don't cram too many clothes into one space. Organize dresser drawers so items are neat and easy to find. If you maintain your wardrobe properly, every item will be ready whenever you need it.

Be sure you are well dressed whenever you go out. Knowing you look your best (even if you're just running errands) will lift your spirits and increase self-confidence. Include colorful items in your wardrobe; they will add energy and interest to your look. Never leave the house if you are unhappy with what you are wearing—it is to your benefit to take an extra minute or two to change and leave in a good mood.

Footwear and Accessories

Every woman loves shoes. The easiest way to gain height instantly is to put on high heels. Heels elongate your feet and make them more attractive. When you walk in heels, remember always to step forward in a straight line from the hip. This will keep your back straight and avoid an unattractive, round-shouldered stance. If you prefer platform shoes, pay attention to the weight and form of the platform—you don't want to give the impression that you are standing on heavy bricks. In the summertime, light gold or natural-colored sandals are essential; these can be combined with any color clothing, and they dizzily extend the foot.

Accessories add the finishing touch to your look, so choose them carefully. Check yourself in the mirror to decide what extra items are appropriate. For example, a necklace or pin might add interest to a simple sweater or jacket. Or you might put on a bracelet that complements your shoes, belt, or bag. Sometimes accessories are used to highlight a certain color in your outfit, but the idea that "everything must match" is definitely a thing of the past.

If you ever need to change your look quickly (perhaps dressing up a business outfit for a dinner date), you can easily replace earrings or add a colorful scarf. It's a good idea to keep spare earrings, a sparkly bracelet, and perhaps some fishnet tights in your handbag so you are prepared whenever the opportunity for an interesting evening arises.

The key to accessorizing well is to accurately pick up accent colors and to use moderation. Be careful, too, when "mixing metals." Some colors lend themselves better to gold or silver. If you choose to use both, however, avoid mixing items in close proximity—a silver necklace and large gold earrings, for example. The same earrings with a silver ring and white gold watch, however, are fine.

Accessorizing should be fun. Put your imagination to work creating an outward image that reflects the personality inside. And do it with great pleasure!

Spend Wisely

Give careful thought to every purchase. Never buy anything just because it is a great bargain. That bargain may hang in your closet for years and your money will be wasted. Everyone likes to save money, but it is better to spend a little more for something you will wear often and enjoy wearing.

Whether you're shopping at Target or a fashionable boutique, the most important consideration in buying a piece of clothing is how well it looks on you. Does it fit perfectly, and is it comfortable? Also consider the quality of materials and workmanship in relation to price. Is it a good value? (And remember, nothing is a good value unless you are sure you will actually wear it.)

Never buy clothing just because it is fashionable—millions of women own fashionable items that have hung, unworn, in their closets for years

If you are thinking of investing in an expensive coat or pair of boots, first determine if this is something you really need and, if so, whether it has classic lines that will always be in style. Once you have decided to spend the money, choose a high-quality item in neutral shades so it can serve you through the years.

If you live in a climate with excessive heat or cold, be sure your seasonal purchases are practical. A winter coat should be both beautiful and warm, and a flirty summer dress may be more comfortable (and versatile) than a halter top and shorts. When buying sunglasses, look for high-quality ones with 100% UVA protection.

Be serious about your purchases. Good clothing can be expensive, and buying clothes you never wear is like throwing money to the wind. If you want a second opinion on items, shop with someone you trust, but do not pay attention to compliments from sales personnel whose earnings may be commission-based. Occasionally we all make purchases we regret; the goal is not to make similar mistakes in the future.

Your clothes make a very visible statement about who you are. Take time to shop wisely and dress well so that statement accurately projects your unique personality.

Your Turn: Sometime when you're feeling good about life in general, take a good look in the mirror. What about your appearance especially appeals to you? Are there any changes you would like to make? Is it time for a new hair color or updated style? Do your eyebrows need shaping, or your cheeks need a blush of color? Be honest, but reasonable. To keep from being too hard on yourself, imagine you are making these suggestions to your best friend instead of yourself.

Now find a comfortable place to sit. Write down whatever changes you are contemplating. If there are more than two items, *prioritize them according to your own criteria (easiest first, most affordable first, most needed first, etc.).*

Once you've decided on physical changes, think about the styles and types of clothes you'd like to see yourself in. Make drawings, write detailed explanations, or cut pictures from magazines. Using these as a guide, add a few specific clothing items to your list.

Finally, clean out your closet to make room for the new clothes you'd like to purchase. Get rid of items that have faded, lost their shape, or have permanent stains. Donate usable pieces that no longer appeal to you. Do not leave anything in the closet that needs repair. If you really love the piece, take it to a seamstress. Otherwise, get rid of it.

All these steps don't have to happen at once. While it's probably a good idea to jot down proposed physical changes while they're fresh in your mind, it's okay (and fun) to take some time developing a portfolio of possible style changes. Do some window shopping to get an idea of costs and determine the best values within your budget. And embrace the opportunity to clean out your closet—you will find your spirits lifted as you revisit pleasant memories, purge the not-so-pleasant ones, and set aside good usable clothing for those in less affluent circumstances. Finally, the extra space you've created will serve as a positive daily reminder of the personal changes you have promised yourself.

Tips for Managing (and Saving) Money

Happiness is not in the mere possession of money; it lies in the joy of achievement, in the thrill of creative effort.   – Franklin D. Roosevelt

Spending money wisely means different things to different people, depending on their personal priorities. Ask yourself, "What is important for me? What are my dreams and how can I best use my money to realize those dreams?" As you spend money, be very aware of whether you are balancing income and expenses. Then ask, "Is my money working for me the way I want it to?" If the answer is "No," you need to create a money management plan, including a realistic budget. Monitor your spending and make adjustments as needed, but discipline yourself to adhere to the basic plan. Be careful that your expenses do not exceed your income. Always think ahead; you have not come to Earth for just a day.

When people think of a budget, they generally think of this much money for rent, that much for food, and so on. Sometimes they forget that an important part of any budget is the money they pay themselves. Each time you receive money, first set aside a percentage for yourself. The amount doesn't matter—one percent or ten percent—what's important is that you do it regularly. Investing in your own dreams will help you achieve your goals.

Another important budget item is a savings plan for any difficult times you may face in the future (serious illness, job loss, etc.). Ideally, that savings should equal about six months' salary.

Be a smart shopper. Watch for sales and/or use coupons for items that you buy regularly. When purchasing expensive items, first check prices in at least three shops. Do some research before buying electronics or a car. Be sure you understand any differences in features, construction quality, or service warranties. Shop with your head, not your heart, and never buy anything just because the price has been deeply discounted. If you don't really need it, it's not a bargain.

Be a smart grocery shopper. Avoid shopping for groceries when you are hungry, because you will nearly always buy items you don't really need. If you purchase items in bulk, be sure you can use them before the quality deteriorates. Otherwise, you are simply throwing money away. Try to shop without children; you will save both time and money. Finally, always check receipts to be sure you have been charged the correct price. If you pay with cash, be sure to count your change.

If you purchase items online, use sites of companies that you know. If a site seems to lack appropriate security, do not provide any personal information. (If the web address is preceded by the letters https, your information should be protected.) When you create a password, use a combination of letters, figures and symbols, and do not use the same password for all sites. Pay attention when typing item codes and quantities; otherwise you may end up with two items when you only wanted one or a green dress when you wanted blue. Keep a copy of the purchase information, including the order or confirmation number.

Credit cards are convenient and popular. However, it is very easy to spend too much money because you don't actually feel the money in your hands when you pay. Be very cautious with these cards; they can get you into big debt very quickly. Cash is the best option for smaller purchases because you can easily see the bills disappearing in your wallet. Debit cards are better than credit, but you need to check your account daily so you know how much money you actually have.

Nowadays many banks offer programs to track your spending online. These can be very helpful in managing expenses. There are also software programs (QuickBooks, for example) that provide complete money management systems. One feature that is especially useful is the comparison of expenses from month to month. Evaluate your current money management skills to decide whether you are fine with a paper and pencil budget or need more sophisticated tools to make your money work for you.

Your Turn: *Most of us have no idea just how much we spend on unnecessary items. For one month, make a detailed list of every purchase and the amount. Use common sense. It's okay to write "Groceries - $75" if all the items are indeed basic foods, cleaning supplies, etc. If, however, $20 of that $75 is spent for wine, a seasonal decoration (Christmas wreath, for example), or other non-grocery purchase, those items should be noted separately. Be sure to record every cent spent—you may be surprised to see how much you're wasting on items that are not really important. Once you know where your* *money is going, it's much easier to create a budget that puts it to better use.*

A Woman's World

Nobody can bring you peace but yourself. – Ralph Waldo Emerson

Self Acceptance

Both outward beauty and inward happiness begin in your mind. To be happy in your own body means being at peace with what you see on the outside and who you are on the inside—your core beliefs, values, and dreams. Do not dwell on imperfections. Focus instead on what makes you unique and special.

Write an affirmation that is appropriate for you at this time in your life. Repeat that affirmation every morning, out loud. (If you don't know what to write, many affirmations are available online. Find one that works, or adapt one to suit your situation.) Most of us wish to feel attractive, successful and appreciated. Accordingly, you should repeat daily: "I am an attractive woman, loved by my husband and children, respected by my peers, and happy. I can be successful in all my endeavors." It is important to believe what you speak; the words must reflect your emotions. Affirmations affect your subconscious, and you will automatically start to achieve results. An affirmation can be created for any sphere of life that interests you or is important to you, but remember to always state your thoughts positively. Never use negative words, even if the thought is positive. For example, do not say "I do not wish to be ill," because "ill" is the strongest word in the affirmation. Instead, say "I want to be healthy." Your thoughts influence your future; therefore you should always think and speak positively.

Never compare yourself to others, as this leads directly to loss of self-esteem and self-confidence. Always try to be realistic—do not belittle yourself or exaggerate your strengths. Trust yourself and your ability to complete tasks. Believe that you have control over your life. Tell yourself every day that you are highly capable and then act according to that belief.

Above all, trust yourself. Don't think of yourself in negative terms or speak badly of yourself, even if people about you may speak unflatteringly. (Again, this doesn't mean you can't be realistic. Telling yourself "I will be on time today" is much more effective than saying "I'm always late.") Love and respect yourself; in response, people surrounding you will treat you the same. If you do not learn to respect yourself, nobody else can do it for you.

Take care of your body. Self-esteem depends on good health. A sound body is necessary for healthy thinking. If your health is poor, little else seems important in life. (Note: There is a difference between good health, which we can control, and disease, like cancer or multiple sclerosis, which we can't. Maintaining good health and fitness can, however, protect us from a number of serious diseases.) Regardless of your outlook and education, remember that it is not selfish to take good care of yourself so that you can also care properly for your family. You set the example for your husband and children; if you do not manage your own health and fitness, how can you teach them good habits?

Family

Some people are polite and accommodating at work, but bossy or complaining at home. It's natural to relax a little when you're at home, but your positive attitude and loving behavior towards family members show how much you love them. Even when you are busy, remember to pay attention to those you love. Respect parents—your own and your husband's. Do not allow them to control your present life, but always make a place for them in your future. Treat them with love and understanding.

Be an active listener in conversations with loved ones. Learn from them; "read" them like you might read a book, soaking up every idea. They are here for you, and you for them. Relationships with family members should be mutually respectful. Try to maintain the same standards of behavior with everyone.

When you disagree with a family member, pause for minute so you can think rationally (not emotionally) and calm down. Be patient. We all know that in most quarrels both people are guilty—remember that. It's also important that no one's feelings are hurt during a conversation, especially if the offended person is a relative. Hurt feelings can last a long time sometimes end up dividing families.

Treat children with tenderness, understanding, gentle but consistent authority, and lots of affection. Take a genuine interest in their lives, and have real conversations with them every day. Let them know that they can depend on your support, your friendship and your advice. Respect their secrets, even if they seem unimportant, remembering how you trusted your parents when you were a child.

It is important to tell your children that you love them. It is not enough to assume they know this; they need to hear you say it. Tell them every day that you love them and that they are precious to you. If you and your children quarrel, or if you must discipline them, never leave them alone until you have reconciled and assured them of your love.

Children also need to know that you are their mother, not one of their playmates. You are strong, you are important, you are the boss. They need to respect you and your opinions, but you must remember that your children also have opinions which you need to consider. Always address children with the same respect you show adults so they will learn to respond in a similar tone.

Teach your children. When they are young, engage them in reading, sports or other outdoor activities, and quiet inside games. Teach them good nutrition and hygiene, so they know how to take care of themselves. Let them help when you prepare meals or clean the house. Teach older ones how to manage their time and money, how to be assertive without being rude, how to listen and communicate effectively. Teach daughters everything you know about cooking, keeping an orderly home, and maintaining quality relationships.

Make your family's health and happiness a top priority. Work diligently to make your home a place where your children (of any age) want to be. Do not allow someone else's beliefs or behaviors to destroy what you have created.

Other Relationships

Have girlfriends who you can laugh with, cry with, share your dreams and fears with—and trust to keep your confidences. Value these friendships. Try not to forget your friends, even when life gets very busy. Wish them a happy birthday and remember them at holidays.

Sometimes it is difficult to distinguish a good person from a person with harmful intentions. The "bad" person smiles and carries on a friendly conversation, and you never think that he or she may be capable of meanness in relation to you. People who are consumed with envy and hatred lose their ability to think reasonably. Be cautious in conversations with strangers or anyone who seems to have these qualities.

If you find yourself with a person who has obviously harmful intentions, end the conversation and remove yourself from the individual. To change their intentions is not within your power, and you need to think first of your own safety (emotional and physical). If this person is a relative, spend as little time with her as possible. Once you are away from the individual, it is important not to dwell on this person or the harm he or she has caused or tried to cause. There are also people who simply wish to have power over you. Do not give it to them. You are in control. You are free to choose how you want to live, and you should not be a pawn in someone else's plan.

Listen to the counsel of people you respect and who would never wish you harm, but treat the counsel of others with caution. Avoid serious conversations with anyone you do not trust. If an acquaintance retells gossip or speaks negatively about someone, be assured that, behind your back, she talks the same way about you.

Do not allow others to humiliate or offend you. You cannot control what others say or how they behave, but you do have complete control over how you respond. Be gracious; nothing is ever gained by sarcasm, put-downs, or demeaning behavior. Do not feel that you must conform to other people's expectations. Politely excuse yourself from people who make you uncomfortable. Spend time with people who like you as you are—people who think and speak honestly and kindly.

Finally, do not try to change others. If you think someone else's life needs changing, consider first how suggesting that change may affect your relationship with her in the future. Trust your instincts.

Your World

In summary, the center of each woman's world is herself—not because she is egotistical, but because her ability to deal with "the world" starts with acceptance of herself. The next sphere of a woman's influence is her family, followed by relationships in general society. The suggestions below reflect ideas that other women have found helpful in maintaining their own sense of personal worth and achieving a balance between their personal, family, and professional roles in society.

Attitude

- *Be happy, consciously savoring each moment of your life. Be grateful for little pleasures.*

- *Think only positive thoughts. Believe that life holds wonderful moments for you.*

Learn something new each day. Open your mind to new ideas.

- *Manage your time wisely. Do not feel you must be busy every minute—balancing rest and relaxation with work and family duties benefits both physical and mental health.*

- *Remember that the past is over, that only what happens from this moment on is important. You can learn from the past, however if you perceive errors as lessons.*

- *Do not always wish that your life was different. Be happy with what you have, but also consider what you can do to make your life better.*

- *Decide what is most important in your life. Then, when you experience disappointment or a sense of hopelessness, focus on that goal or item of importance until you regain your perspective.*

- *Focus your thoughts on positive people—people who are generous and helpful or who make your own life better. Do not waste thoughts on people who are negative.*

- *Do not fear those who speak ill of you. Instead, learn to transform their negative energy into motivational power for yourself.*

- *Do not spend too much time worrying about how you look, how you should change, or what others think of you. Do, however, pay attention to how others respond to you. If acquaintances tend to lose their smiles while visiting with you, perhaps you need to be a bit more positive. It's alright to share problems with friends, but be sure to also share the good times. Listen to what people tell you and respond to their experience before sharing your own. Don't be a complainer; if you always complain, your friends will assume that you complain about them to others.*

- *Remember that sometimes it is easier to change yourself in relation to the rest of the world than to change the whole world.*

Behavior

- *Show love to children, animals, to plants and everything that surrounds you.*
- *Always use gracious expressions such as "please," "thank you," and "I'm sorry." Good manners are always in fashion, so it is wise to practice them.*
- *Never use vulgar or abusive expressions. Be positive with others, and smile. (If necessary, practice before a mirror until it becomes natural.)*
- *Include some physical activity in every day.*
- *Think before speaking so you do not say anything silly or hurtful.*
- *Always think carefully before saying something about someone else. You don't want to damage their reputation or your own. Be fair; treat others as you want them to treat you. Be trustworthy with secrets.*
- *When things do not go as you had hoped or planned, stop and think for a minute. Perhaps this is a situation where it is easier, and better, to simply go with the flow.*

- *Try not to appear anxious, even if you are frustrated or in a hurry. Be calm and self-assured. Walk gracefully, as though you are taking part in a fashion show.*

- *It is natural to become sad, angry, and frustrated when we are sick or going through a difficult period in life. But do not let pain or difficulty become fear. Do not worry over things you cannot change. Accept what cannot be changed, work through what can; and then move on.*

- *Keep a smile on your public face. If you've had a bad day, people around you don't need to know about it. Never bare your soul to the first person who comes along. Share disappointments and heartaches only with close friends or relatives.*

- *Always try to look as good as possible. Save baggy pants and tennis shoes for the gym, and take an extra minute to apply lipstick before running an errand. Remember that you are a woman—wear clothing and accessories that appropriately reflect your femininity.*

- *Keep your home tidy, clean, and cozy. Think of it as a nest filled with love, a safe haven for your family, and your favorite place to be.*

- *If you find yourself in a bad situation, try to find a way to turn it around (to make sweet lemonade from sour lemons).*

As you practice these attitudes and behaviors, you will learn to love and respect your inner self, and life will become easier. Decisions regarding serious problems will come to you, and you will trust your intuition and act accordingly.

Your Turn: Reread the bulleted lists regarding attitude and behavior. Place a check or ☺ next to items you are already doing. Review the remaining ones and choose one item to focus on for the next month. At the end of the month, decide if you have successfully integrated that attitude or behavior. If so, add a check or ☺ with the date and choose another item (preferably from the other list) to work on the following month.

Defining Success, and Achieving It

*Always bear in mind that your own resolution to succeed is
more important than any other. – Abraham Lincoln*

Anything you can imagine, you can also make come true. Broaden your range of interests, step forward with head held high, and make grand plans for your future without worrying about what others may say.

Decide for yourself what you desire from life and how you define success. Say to yourself, "This is what I want to achieve. No one else can give me success. I must take charge of my own life to make this happen." If you do not know what you want, make time for whatever will allow you to step outside yourself and take a detached view of your life. For some, this may mean lots of quiet time in bookstores, museums or other reflective places. Some may immerse themselves in crowds and conversation, drawing ideas from others in order to distill their own. Some will seek adventure, pushing themselves to physical limits. And some will find a one-on-one conversation with a life coach or other counselor to be most helpful.

Inside each of us is a little GPS voice telling us what turns are ahead and how to correct our course when we've missed a turn. Listen to that voice—it will lead you to success. Don't trust your life to chance; create your own good fortune. Success is within your reach. Live the best life you can. You control your destiny.

Set specific goals, both long- and short-term, and consistently work toward those. Every day, do something—no matter how small—that brings you closer to your dream. Make the most of today because tomorrow may not provide the same opportunity. If you make a wrong turn along the way, be sure to begin your correction course the very next day. Protect your reputation; be a person of integrity. If you have promise something, it is important that you do it.

People who achieve financial independence are engaged in work they enjoy. Try to engage yourself in things that not only bring pleasure but also complement your talents and fulfill your dreams. Open your mind to new ideas and experiences. Always be striving to learn or try something new. Read books, talk to people about what you are learning, and don't be afraid to ask questions.

Seek a mentor within your expanding world—a smart, successful woman who shares some of your aspirations and/or talents. Talk with this woman; study her habits; discuss possible variants of your own future and the best path to your ultimate dream.

Each year provides only 8760 hours. Most of us sleep through about a thousand of those, but we need to make conscious decisions about how we spend the rest. Lay out your goals, make a plan, and operate according to that plan. It's really very simple. Don't obsess over time, but always be aware of it. Consciously choose the best, most productive way to spend it. Ask yourself, "What is important to me? What best serves my future goals?" If necessary, be ready (and willing) to change your plan. Continue to monitor your choices with questions: "Is this what I want?" "Is this the best way to achieve my goal?"

Remember that the secret of a woman's strength is knowledge of what she wants and how to achieve it. Lay each goal before you and work toward it. When you reach that goal, lay out a new one. Never feel that there is nothing more to be achieved; life without goals becomes stagnant. Make the best use of every opportunity life affords you; be afraid of nothing. Trust in your dream even if others doubt— it's your resolution to succeed that produces results.

__Your Turn:__ Make a list of 100 things you want to do during your lifetime. They can be as big as running your own business or as small as planting a flower. Have you always longed to visit France, take ballet lessons, or play the piano? Do you want to build something, grow something, or write something? Write your wish list, post it where you will see it every day, and start living your dreams!

Afterword

A Woman's World is for every woman who wishes to carry herself with the style and confidence of a movie star, to live comfortably within her means, be a favorite among family and friends, and achieve success in whatever endeavors she chooses. Within these pages I have revealed the unique secrets of female success. If you have enjoyed the Your Turn activities, you are already on the path of positive change that fosters success. Now it is up to you to stay on the path by continuing these habits.

Every day, life gives us hundreds of opportunities to change our lives for the better. Learn to recognize these opportunities; then use them as starting points to achieve your own goals. Seize the day—live each moment to the fullest, and never forget that the life is a gift.

Take control of your life. Discover your deepest dream and make it happen. Do not put it off, and do not get sidetracked. Do something right now to achieve it. Set aside negative fears. Think only positive thoughts—acting on those will move you forward. Determine what you really want from life and, using this book as a guide, develop and follow a plan to reach the goals you have laid out.

Mark Twain put it this way: "Twenty years from now you will more disappointed by the things you didn't do than by the ones you did do. So catch the trade winds in your sails. Explore. Dream. Discover." Good luck as you set sail on your future. Be happy and enjoy the voyage!

Thanks to my husband Michael, my son Nikolay, and my daughter Olesya for their never-ending love, understanding, and support of my dreams. I love you very much.

To my parents, Sergey and Galina, to my sister Oksana and her family, and to my friends for believing in me and pushing me forward. I love you all.

Thanks to my great editor, Alison Miller, who has helped me throughout this project. It has been a joy working with her.

Thanks also to Ylyana Shershunova for the picture on the page #9. Her sweet personality and wonderful artistic talent are very inspiring.

Many thanks to everyone who made this happen. It has been an amazing experience.